NATURAL REMEDIES FOR HYPERTENSION / HIGH BLOOD PRESSURE

- NUTRITIONAL REMEDIES SERIES -

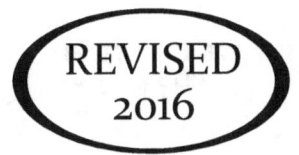

REVISED
2016

T. A. SHOBUKOLA

i

ISBN   1981452323

ISBN 978-1981452323
2016

DEDICATION

This book is dedicated to the glory of God the Giver of life and the creator of the universe and all that is in it.

I am highly grateful to Him for the inspiration and the wisdom to put this small effort together. May all Praise and Honour be His for ever. Amen.

ACKNOWLEDGEMENT

I wish to register my deep appreciation to all who had contributed to the success of this publication in one way or the other , those who had offered useful information and assistance in various ways, especially, the various authors whose works had been copiously quoted or cited.

May the God Almighty bless them all abundantly. Particularly , I thank God for The book of books , The Holy Bible.

FOREWORD

This small book is my humble contribution in revealing the salient and usually unknown   fatal danger of this disease ,High Blood Pressure ,dubbed the "Silent killer".

I had earlier written a few pages on this ailment in my book, "NUTRITIONAL   REMEDIES FOR COMMO N AILMENTS" but I was prompted in to further reading and researching on it after I was suddenly stuck by this ailment. I studied to gather all the information I could find on the topic, along with the available natural/ home remedies for it in order provide quality information for people who may want to improve their quality of life and avoid the "Silent killer".

I jokingly promised friends that I will expose hypertension to the whole world for daring to strike me. This book is therefore the fulfillment of the promise.

This is   with the optimum aim of raising the awareness of majority of people to the need to be watchful and careful of this ailment which is said to affect more than one billion people world-wide because it has neither a geographical nor demographical barrier; it respects neither race nor age.

The cheering news as my research had shown is that as dangerous as hypertension is, it can be overcome with natural remedies through simple change in diet and life-style,without resorting to medication or drugs with the usual attendant dangerous side- effects.

In fact Natural cure for hypertension is the most effective and potent remedy for normalizing high blood pressure. Synthetic medications only lower the heart rate or only ease the pressure on the arteries while   natural remedies actually cure the problem from the arteries, it is therefore the key to a healthy livi

INTRODUCTION

High blood pressure also known as hypertension is a disease of the modern age . The fast pace of life coupled with the mental and physical pressure as a result of the increasingly industrialized and metropolitan environment which make it almost impossible to live a stress-free life play a major role in the rising cases of high blood pressure.

It is commonly called "The silent killer" because it usually strikes unnoticed , due to lack of symptoms in most cases. A lot of dangerous health problems are created if left untreated ; it is therefore highly advisable for everyone to ascertain his/her blood pressure status regularly.

This book provides almost all you need to know about this dreaded ailment in a layman terms : how your blood pressure can be measured , the possible causes of both the essential and secondary hypertension,   common risk factors and how to avoid them, life style and diet changes and the relevance of physical exercise .It provides ten simple and suitable tips on physical exercise you can do to lower your blood pressure without interfering   with your daily responsibilities and commitments, it lists the effect of stress and gives ten simple methods to manage it and live a stress-free life. Forty-two simple and natural ways to cure high blood pressure are also discussed. Also included are several hypertension diet tips.

It had been said that of all the countless debilitating and harmful ailments, high blood pressure is one of the easiest to prevent and one of the most responsive to natural treatment. All the recommendations in this book will help you to lower your high blood pressure naturally and if you have normal blood pressure it will help you from developing high blood pressure. You will also find answer to ten frequently   Asked Questions [FQA] on hypertension in the book.

Disclaimer

The book, "NATURAL REMEDIES FOR HYPERTENSION HIGH BLOOD PRESSURE" had been written as a practical health guide. Every effort had been made to make this report as complete and accurate as possible. However, there may be mistakes in typography or contents It contains information on hypertension home remedies for those who want to avail themselves of the abundant God-given natural Remedies for human health.

It is solely for informational purposes and may be used with the advice of your physician or health care provider.

CONTENTS

CHAPTER ONE

AN OVERVIEW

High blood Pressure, also called hypertension is a health disorder in which the blood pressure in the arteries remains higher than normal. Naturally blood pressure is the force by which the heart pumps blood into the blood arteries, blood vessels, throughout the human body under a certain pressure. Blood pressure rises and falls throughout the day; it goes up during physical exercise or while doing serious brain work or when one is excessively worried and comes down later   but when it stays elevated over time , it is called high blood pressure.

There are two types of hypertension ;
The essential hypertension which is often referred to simply as high blood pressure. Also known as primary hypertension, has no clear cause and is thought to be linked to genetics, poor diet, lack of exercise and obesity Secondary hypertension is high blood pressure that is caused by another medical Conditions that affect the arteries, heart or endocrine system. It is also is caused by an underlying disease such as diabetes or kidney problems.It can also occur during pregnancy, Eclampsia.

•   High blood pressure is dangerous because it puts strain on the heart and the circulatory system ; if left untreated can ultimately cause heart failure, heart attack, hardening of the arteries, stroke , kidney disease,Diabetes, vision loss, metabolic syndromeand other cardiovascular diseases. It is a very dangerous and sometimes life-threatening condition which knows no race or geographical barrier, affecting people all around the world.

High blood pressure often has no signs or symptoms hence it is known as "The silent killer". Since several factors and conditions play a role, it is difficult to identify a specific cause , even the health care profession does not claim to know the cause of high blood pressure.

However, there are a lot of factors that contribute to it; these include but not limited to smoking, lack of physical activity, obesity, high sodium in-take, high cholesterol, excessive consumption of alcohol and of course heredity. Diabetic patients are also at greater risk of developing high blood pressure. Many of the risk factors can be controlled before it gets dangerously high. High blood pressure does not discriminate, it can happen to any one at any age.

Normal   Blood
pressure
Blood pressure itself is not a disease that needs to be cured, the right level of pressure is needed to circulate the blood throughout the body. It does need however to be controlled to

avoid a condition of low pressure, called hypotension , that is too low and deprives the body of oxygen and nutrients or high blood pressure called hypertension, that is too high and strains the heart and the blood vessels.

Blood pressure is measured with the aid of a Digital blood pressure Monitor, called Sphygmomanometer, which comes in different sizes, shapes and makes. The blood pressure measurement is recorded in two readings-the systolic and the diastolic readings. The former ,which is on top , records the pressure when the hearts contracts and pumps out the blood while the latter, which is below , records the reading when the heart is relaxed and is filled with blood.

Below is a table classifying blood pressure values in accordance with the World Health Organization{ WHO} Records.   This could be used for reference purposes.

Range	Systolic [mmHg]	Diastolic [mmHg]
Hypotension	Less 100	Less 60
Normal Pressure	120-139	80-89
Mild Hypertension	140-159	90-99
Moderately serious	160-179	100-109
Serious Hypertension	180 and above	110 and above

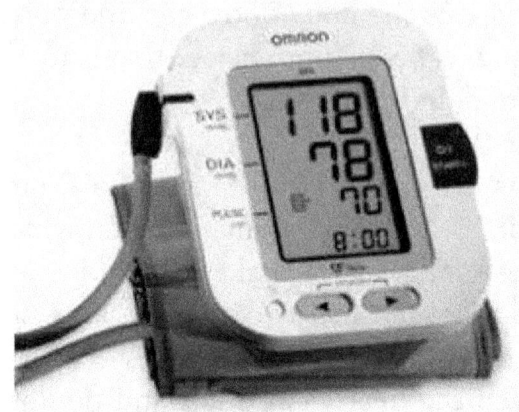

A Sphygmomanometer- A typical Blood Pressure Monitor

Chapter Two

CAUSES OF HYPERTENSION

The exact causes of high blood pressure are not known, but several factors and conditions may contribute to its development Hypertension, also known as high blood pressure, is a major risk factor for both heart attacks and strokes. According to the American Heart Association, almost
75 million people have hypertension. Many factors contribute to high blood pressure , among these are genetics, stress, a sedentary lifestyle , poor diet.

Stress

.

The hustle and bustle of daily life in our urban cities impact adversely on human health; rising from bed in the wee hour of the day to get ready for the day, getting oneself ready for work and the children for school is highly demanding; having to leave home early to beat the early morning traffic rush whether you are driving or taking public transport makes no difference, added is the struggle through the over congested traffic on home-ward journey. The problem becomes more complex if you have to rush to pick up the kids from school or day-care centre only to get home late and still have to go through the normal domestic chores, ending up going late to bed and rising up early without sufficient rest the next   day to continue the usual   daily   routine.   The   daily   personal   church responsibilities   or   social   commitments   cannot   also   be neglected.

The pressure of meeting the set target at work ,either employed or   self-employed in order to make ends meet is also always present. Included   is the care , worry and anxiety of cost of leaving, the ever soaring cost of food stuff , transportation and general cost of living in this age of global economic meltdown are also always there to worry about.

Worry for security of life and property and unstable source of electric power supply   and   fuel coupled with   the ever disturbing perennial noise of generators, from the big industrial type to the proliferation of the "I-better-my-neighbour" type
,during the day and night have their tolls on the health
also
The list seems inexhaustible as you will realize from your daily personal experience.

Executive
stress:
Care and worry of getting the organization going ,working round the clock without a definite closing time and stuffing the tummy with denatured food like snacks , sodium -rich fast food and sugar-loaded drinks such as soft drinks and synthetic fruit juices , coordinating   the efforts of the various units and departments   all to ensure the company

remains afloat in the

face of the global economic melt-down are few of the causes of the executive stress .

Emotional
stress:

Stress definitely affects our body; in addition to the emotional discomfort we feel when faced with stressful situation, our bodies react by releasing tress hormones (adrenalin and cortisol) into the blood to prepare the body for the "fight or light" response .This makes the heart to beat faster and constrict the blood vessel in order to get more blood to the core of the body instead of the extremities. The constriction of the vessels and increase in heart pulse raise the blood pressure, but only temporarily ,because the pressure returns to its pre- stress level when the stress reaction goes away. However, our modern society contains a lot of stressful   events ; such chronic/constant stress causes the body to be under constant stress for days and weeks at times. This may well be the link between stress and high blood pressure.

Emotional stress makes the blood arteries to constrict and thereby makes the blood pressure to rise. Chronic anger and hostility have strong effect on the blood pressure. Learn to be at peace with God and men at all times.

Overweight
.

Blood pressure often increases as weight increases. Losing just

10 pounds (4.5 kilograms) can help reduce your blood pressure.

In general, the more weight you lose, the lower your blood pressure. Losing weight also makes any blood pressure medications one is taking to be more effective.

Besides shedding pounds, you should also keep an eye on your waistline. Carrying too much weight around your waist can put you at greater risk of high blood pressure. In general: Men are at risk if their waist measurement is greater than 40 inches (102 centimeters, or cm). Women are at risk if their waist measurement is greater than 35 inches (89 cm). Asian men are at risk if their waist measurement is greater than 36 inches (91 cm). Asian women are at risk if their waist measurement is greater than 32 inches (81 cm).

Maintaining a reasonable weight is important to minimize the risk of several major diseases, including high blood pressure. For overweighed people even a small weight loss can dramatically reduce or even prevent high blood pressure. This is not unconnected with the fact that the heart will not have to work as hard. In losing weight it is important to do it gradually; it had been advised that not more than 2 pounds should be lost weekly. This is the healthiest way to lose weight that offers the best chance of long-term success.

There is usually no magic approach or formula for weight loss; just eat fewer calories than is needed for normal daily activities because it is not only what is eaten that adds calories but also how much. It is usually recommended that some water be taken before meal to reduce the quantity of food consumed.

Take note of the following calories-saving hints:

- Use low fat or fat –free condiments, such as fat free salad dressings.
- Eat smaller food portions ,cut back gradually.
- Choose low fat or fat-free diary products to reduce total fat in-take.
- Avoid food with lots of added sugar such as ice cream, candy-bars, soft drinks and synthetic fruit juices
- Eat fruits and vegetables in their natural forms.
- Drink plenty of water.

It is best to work out some combination of both eating less and being more physically active for an effective weight loss programme.

Too much common salt in the diet.

Reducing salt intake is one of the quickest ways to reduce the blood pressure, particularly if one already has it.

A high salt diet disrupts the natural sodium balance in the body. This causes fluid retention which increases the pressure exerted by the blood against blood vessel walls (high blood pressure). For every one gram of salt we cut from our average daily intake, there would be fewer deaths from strokes and heart attacks each year

Lack of physical exercise.

Exercise regularly: Ensure physical activity and avoid sedentary work

Being physically active is one of the most important things one can do to prevent or control high blood pressure. This is contrary to the general belief of some that a hypertensive person should always be resting or taking it easy.

A single exercise session can lower the blood pressure by 5 to 7 mmHg. Risk factors are increased when added weight is in the abdominal area of the body. It should be noted that it does not take much effort to be physically active; all that is needed is just about 30 minutes which may be sub-divided into shorter periods of at least 10 minutes each, of moderate-level physical activity on most days of the week.

Listed below are some examples of such activities:
- Brisk walking/strolling
- Bicycling
- Gardening/Raking of leaves.
- Washing and Waxing of a car
- Washing of window panes or floors.
- Lawn mowerring
- Stair –walking, up and down.
- Using the stair case in lieu of the elevator
- Dropping off from a bus one or two bus stops and trek

down to one's destination.

➤ Parking one's car at the far end of the parking lot at
     the
   place of work.

Smoking
.

Tobacco use is the most common cause of avoidable cardiovascular mortality worldwide.Smoking causes an acute increase in blood pressure (BP) and heart rate and has been found to be associated with malignant hypertension.
It has a detrimental effect on the circulatory system. It acutely elevates the blood pressure level; it increases the systolic count by at least 20mm Hg. It is also found to be an independent factor in complicating renal function through elevating high blood pressure.

Old
age.
The older   one gets the   greater the likelihood of developing hypertension. This is due to arteriosclerosis (hardening of the artery walls)   It is said that people inclined to hypertension usually begin to show the symptoms in their early thirties.

Alcohol
consumption.
Drinking too much alcohol can raise the blood pressure with many other harmful effects to the body. Alcohol also contains calories, which matter particularly if one needs to

lose weight.

Family history.

Family history and genetics do have roles in hypertension. Those with family history of high blood pressure are much likely to develop it than others. It is known that children in families prone to high blood pressure usually have the tendency towards the sickness. The following questions are relevant to

help you ascertain your risk level;

- Family history of cardiovascular disease ?
- Hardy relative experienced a stroke or stroke symptoms?
- Any family history of diabetes?
- Does family life style predisposes it to hypertension?

Chapter Three

SYMPTOMS OF HIGH BLOOD PRESSURE.

High blood pressure is often called the "Silent Killer" because It has no symptoms and goes undetected for years unless the pressure is checked regularly. While it is easy to overlook some of the generally "quiet" signs , the following are some of such clues that can alert one of the problem:

- Occasiona feeling of nausea.
- Dizziness.
- Headache.
- Blurred vision.
- urinating. Frequent and fatigue
- Tiredness
- Poor concentration
- Poor mental health

Unfortunately, these symptoms are common to many other health problems, so the best way is to have a regular check.

POTENTIAL DANGER OF UNTREATED HIGH BLOOD PRESSURE.

Stroke

Uncontrolled hypertension can result in a stroke, Which is

a

damage to the brain due to either a blockade in blood flow or loss of blood from blood vessels in the brain. This blockade or loss of blood flow causes lack of oxygen and needed blood nutrient to the brain. The degree of damage to the brain is dependent on where and how much blood flow to the brain is interrupted.

Heart attack.

The blood vessels can become stiffened or narrowed down leading to blockage of blood flow and a possible heart attack or heart failure in a more severe cases

Impaired vision

Along with causing heart and kidney problems, untreated high blood pressure can also affect your eyesight and lead to eye disease It can cause damage to the blood vessels in the retina, the area at the back of the eye where images focus. This eyedisease is known as hypertensive retinopathy. The damage can be serious if hypertension is not treated

Kidney failure.

Kidneys are supplied with dense blood vessels, and high volumes of blood flow through them. Over time, uncontrolled high blood pressure can cause arteries around the kidneys to narrow, weaken or harden. These damaged arteries are not able to deliver enough blood to the kidney tissue; as more arteries become blocked and stop functioning, the kidneys eventually fail. This process can happen over several years, but it can be prevented.

Sudden
death
The body system can suddenly pack up during an activity or during sleep or rest.

Chapter
Four

ANSWERS TO SOME COMMON FREQUENTLY ASKED QUESTIONS [FAQ] ON HYPERTENSION

Q. What is hypertension?

A: Hypertension is the abnormally high blood pressure (the blood pressure in the arteries) .This is indicated by blood pressure readings of 140mmHg and above (for systolic pressure)(and 90mm Hg and above for the diastolic pressure); all measured while at rest .

Q: How often do I need to measure my blood pressure ?

A: The older one gets ,the more regularly the need for it in order to ensure proper monitoring

Q: What causes High blood pressure?

A: For the majority of people with high blood pressure the causes are not known, but some of the following factors may be responsible: such as over weight, old age, consumption of excess table salt, smoking, lack of exercise, genetics, alcohol consumption, stress.

Q: Which risk Factors contribute to hypertension?

A: These include high sodium[salt] in- take ,sedentary life style, stress, heredity, smoking, alcohol.

Q: Does hypertension affect my sex life?

A: No, once natural remedies are used. Some of the known natural remedies like Ginger, Ginkgo Biloba ,Water melon and COQ10 are known to have aphrodisiac properties . It is only many   prescribed hypertension   drugs   that are linked to erectile dysfunction.

In fact sex is said to have some beneficial effects. According to Joy Davidson , aNew York psychologist and sex Therapist, "sex does a body good in many ways ; the benefits are not just anecdotal or hear-say but backed up by scientific scrutiny:"

Sex lowers blood pressure and   helps over-all stress
reduction, according to a report in the Scotland journal
"Biological Psychology".

Another report in the journal stated that it is associated

with lower diastolic blood pressure.

➢ Yet another research found a link between partner hugs
and lower blood pressure in women.

➢ Also according to a Los Angeles sexologist "Sex is a great mode of exercise" She said that it takes work from both a physical and psychological perspective to do it well.

➢ It is also said that research had shown that it reduces the
risk of fatal heart attacks in men ,by half.

➢ It is also known that it boosts the immune system and
maintain a healthy weight.

Q: How can I measure my blood pressure at home?

A: This can be done by acquiring the blood pressure Monitor.
It helps to eliminate "white coat hypertension" which one may develop when measured by the health provider.

Q: Which are the food high in sodium ?

A: High sodium food consists of processed foods such as sausage ,bacon, canned soup, condiments(ketchup, salad dressings.), fast foods , snacks, popcorn, peanuts. Most processed foods are really high in sodium, even though you may not consider them as salty foods.

Q: Can pregnancy increase blood pressure?

A: Some women develop high blood pressure during pregnancy which usually returns to normal after delivery. This is called pre-eclampsia or toxemia. It is a disorder that occurs only during pregnancy. It is characterized by high blood pressure and elevated protein in the urine, it is dangerous as it can cause fetal complications. When it produces symptoms(not all women have symptoms) they may include swelling oedema, sudden weight gain, headaches and changes in vision.

These are some risk factors:
- Have high blood pressure before pregnancy
- Had developed high blood pressure or pre-eclampsia in previous pregnancy
- Obese prior to pregnancy
- Under 20 or over 40 years old
- Have diabetes, kidney disease or rheumatoid arthritis

Q: how do I know if I am overweight?

A. Overweight is measured in Body Mass Index [BMI]
To compute your BMI, multiply your weight in pounds by 703; then divide the result by the square of your height in inches{ wt.(lbs)x703}
{Ht.(ins) 2 }

A healthy weight is in the range of 18.5 to 24.9 ; overweight is in the range of 25 to 29.

Q: what is the relationship between high blood pressure and cardiovascular disease

A: There is a strong link between the two. This is because the extra work the heart must do to pump the blood round the body will eventually takes its toll on the heart and the arteries. High blood pressure creates a build-up in the arteries and therefore damages them. This as a result greatly increases the risk of cardiovascular disease .

Chapter
Five

SOME HOME REMEDIES
FOR HYPERTENSION

Natural cures for hypertension are the most effective approach to normalize high blood pressure. This is highly necessary in order to avoid the miserable side effects associated with medication.

The mostly recommended method of preventing hypertension is making positive changes in lifestyle .Physical activity, weight reduction, dietary sodium reduction, potassium supplementation, and consumption of a diet rich in fruits, vegetables, and low-fat dairy products, along with reductions in saturated and total fat, have been recommended as effective approaches for the prevention of hypertension.

Some known adverse side effects of using drugs for high blood pressure include ,but not limited to ,rapid heartbeat, heart failure, depression ,fatigue , sexual impotence ,fluid retention, gastrointestinal problems, dizziness, muscle weakness and especially cramping, lowering of good cholesterol, dryness of the mouth, fever, anemia, stuffy nose, diarrhea, heartburn and joint pains .

They are said to also promote the excretion of some helpful minerals like calcium and magnesium from the body. These two minerals have been shown to be effective in lowering elevated blood pressure and to aid in preventing heart attack.

Often the side effects are so bad that other medication with their attendant side effects will be needed to counteract them! Natural remedies work by treating the main problem inside the arteries.

The healthiest diet is a high fiber diet that contains whole grains, fruits, vegetables and lean meats. Fiber is critical for flushing the body of toxins, cholesterol, and plaque build-up. It had also been shown that most people who suffer from high blood pressure are deficient in three key minerals ,namely, Magnesium, Potassium and Calcium which are critical for normalized blood pressure. These can be found in food .

Sources of Magnesium are legumes, whole grains, cereals, nuts, dark green vegetables and cocoa, while those of Potassium are green leafy vegetables, celery, spinach, cabbage, carrots, graps, bananas, potatoes, melon , peas, peppers, pears, tomatoes, water melon and Calcium can be obtained from all green vegetables, carrot, onions, cheese and beans

SOME TOP SUPERFOODS GOOD FOR LOWERING HIGH BLOOD PRESSURE

Many people use prescription medicines to lower blood pressure but one can do the same thing naturally by simply eating the right foods. A healthy diet is one of the most powerful ways to lower blood pressure. Many super-foods can reduce blood pressure in as little as two weeks. Also, these super-foods can lower blood cholesterol, improve sleep and reduce headaches.

Almonds

Nuts like almonds provide protein and healthy fats that are good for your health. The high amount of good protein in almonds and almond milk helps lower high blood pressure and fight against diabetes and cardiovascular disease. The monounsaturated fats in almonds have been found to lower cholesterol levels, reduce arterial inflammation, and ultimately lower blood pressure. The American Heart Association notes that the potassium present in almonds can reduce the negative effects of sodium on blood pressure. Healthy fats also promote cardiovascular health.

Olive Oil

Olive oil has free radical-fighting antioxidants known as polyphenols. These polyphenols help reduce blood pressure by protecting LDL ("bad") cholesterol from oxidation. When too much oxidation of LDL occurs in the blood vessels, they can

become rigid and in turn increase blood pressure. Olive oil also is high in monounsaturated fatty acids like oleic acid, which helps prevent high blood pressure. However, it is essential to bear in mind that olive oil loses much of its health benefits when heated. Due to this, try to use olive oil without cooking it. You can drizzle it on a salad or stir it into a bowl of roasted potatoes to enjoy maximum benefits."Olive oil intake is inversely associated with both systolic and diastolic blood pressure." Consuming more olive oil is linked with lowered blood pressure.

Potatoe
s

Potatoes are rich in potassium and another blood pressure-lowering compound called kukoamines. They also contain an assortment of minerals and vitamins, such as vitamins C, B6, B1 and B3; magnesium, iron, zinc and phosphorus; as well as carotenoids and natural phenols. All these minerals and vitamins are good for your overall health. For best results, be sure to prepare your potatoes without frying them and eat them without adding butter, margarine or sour cream.

Salmo
n

The omega-3 fatty acids as well as EPA (eicosapentaenoic acid), primarily found in cold-water fish like salmon, reduce inflammation and prevent high blood pressure. Also, salmon has low fat and high protein content that is good for people with high blood pressure. Along with salmon, you can also eat other cold-water fishes such as mackerel, halibut, anchovies, tuna, and herring. If you do not like the taste of salmon or other fish, you can take fish oil supplements.

Spinac
h

Spinach is a foliate-rich food that can lower your risk of hypertension. This leafy green vegetable also provides a completely absorbable, balanced protein along with antioxidants that help lower blood pressure. A study published in the Journal of the American Medical Association found that those who consumed at least 1,000 micrograms of spinach foliate a day had a lower risk of hypertension compared with those who consumed 200 micrograms a day. Other good sources of folate-rich foods include legumes and asparagus.

Tomatoe
s

Tomatoes contain lycopene, an antioxidant that helps protect your cells from the damaging effects of free radicals. The lycopene and other carotenoids found in tomatoes help in reducing high blood pressure and lowering the risk of heart disease. Tomatoes also contain nutrients such as calcium, potassium, and vitamins A, C and E that are good for your overall health. A 2006 study published in the American Heart Journal found that regular consumption of 250mg of tomato extract for eight weeks can significantly lower both systolic and diastolic blood pressure among those who have hypertension.

Pomegranate

Pomegranates not only are dense in nutrients, but are also high in antioxidants-specifically in tannins and anthocyanins. Pomegranates are fruits that have a hard shell and edible juicy red seeds. Pomegranates contain phytochemicals, flavonoids, polyphenols, and punicalagin.Phytochemicals naturally occur in plant foods that act as antioxidants and prevent damage to our cells. Antioxidants such as flavonoids and polyphenols fight against heart disease and cancers.Punicalagin is a compound that is mostly responsible for the health benefits in pomegranates. It improves the functions of the heart and blood vessels, lowers bad (LDL) cholesterol, raises good (HDL) cholesterol, lowers high blood pressure, and reverses the effects of arterial blockage (atherosclerosis).Pomegranates contain more antioxidants than red wine, berries, or even green tea.Add pomegranate seeds to your salad, or juice the seeds into a tasty drink.

Beets & Radishes

Beets & radishes are under-appreciated and overlooked vegetables. Both beets and radishes are high in nitrates, which are great at lowering high blood pressure, by improving vasodilation.Nitrates change into vasodilator nitric oxide after being ingested. Nitric acid dilates blood vessels, regulates blood pressure, decreases endothelial inflammation, and platelet aggregation.Both the leaves and the roots of the radish lowers elevated blood pressures. Juice made out of beets or radishes are the best form of the vegetables, in lowering blood pressure.

Drink a glass of blended beets or radishes juice, daily. Also, add fresh beets and radishes to any dish!

HERBS AND SPICES POTENT FOR BLOOD PRESSURE CONTROL.

Basi
l
Basil is a delicious herb that goes well in a variety of foods. It is originally native to Iran, India, and other tropical regions of Asia, but now it is widely available throughout the world. Basil has antioxidant, anti-mutagenic, anti-tumorigenic, anti-viral, and anti-bacterial properties. It also helps lower your blood pressure. Extract of basil has been shown to lower blood pressure.
Basil is a delicious herb that goes well in a variety of foods. It also might help lower your blood pressure. Extract of basil has been shown to lower blood pressure, although only briefly. Keep a small pot of the herb in your garden and add the fresh leaves to pastas, soups, salads, and casseroles.

Cinnamo
n
Cinnamon is another tasty seasoning that requires little effort to include in your daily diet, and it may bring your blood pressure numbers down. Consuming cinnamon every day has been shown to lower blood pressure in people with diabetes. Include more cinnamon in your diet by sprinkling it on your breakfast cereal, oatmeal, and even in your coffee. At dinner, cinnamon enhances the flavor of stir-fries,

curries, and

stews.Cinnamon is another tasty seasoning that requires little effort to include in your daily diet and that may bring your blood pressure numbers down.Cinnamon combined with magnesium, diet, and lifestyle changes may lead to overall reductions in blood pressure up to 25mm Hg.. Include more cinnamon in your diet by sprinkling it on your breakfast cereal .

Cardamo
m

Cardamom is a seasoning that comes from India and is often used in the foods of South Asia. A study investigating the health effects of cardamom found that participants given powdered cardamom daily for several months saw significant reductions in their blood pressure readings. You can include cardamom seeds or the powder in spice rubs, in soups and stews, and even in baked goods for a special flavor and a positive health benefit.

Flaxsee
d

Flaxseed is rich in omega-3 fatty acids, which have been found to lower blood pressure significantly. Flaxseed may protect against atherosclerotic cardiovascular disease by reducing serum cholesterol, improving glucose tolerance and acting as an antioxidant. You can buy many products that contain flaxseed, but a better bet is to buy ground flaxseed or grind it yourself in a coffee grinder and add it to your home cooked meals. The best part about flaxseed is that it can be stirred into virtually any dish, from soups to smoothies to baked goods. Store flaxseed in your freezer for optimum potency.

Ginger

It is another potent remedy for high blood pressure that aids in reducing blood lipids and platelet aggregation .It has also been shown to reduce peripheral resistance in the capillary beds as well as increase capillary permeability. Ginger is a natural blood thinner and therefore may help to prevent stroke, heart attacks and hardening of the arteries . The chemical gingerol in ginger appears to inhibit an enzyme that causes cells to clot and thereby reduces platelet aggregation and blood "clumping". Ginger does not only help fight heart attacks and strokes , but also beneficial in preventing Alzheimer's disease .Ginger is also said to help increase blood circulation, including peripheral circulation (hands, feet, e

Hawthor

n

Hawthorn is an herbal remedy for high blood pressure that has been used in traditional Chinese medicines for thousands of years. Decoctions of hawthorn seem to have a whole host of benefits on cardiovascular health, including reduction of blood pressure, the prevention of clot formation, and an increase in blood circulation. You can take hawthorn as a pill, a liquid extract, or a tea.

Celery

A time-tested Chinese remedy for high blood pressure is celery juice, which can be made with a blender or a juicer. Two to three 8 oz glasses a day for a month can help prevent high blood pressure or restore it to normal. Studies have found that this stalk is packed with over a dozen anti-inflammatory agents, similar to some anti- inflammatory drugs. This crunchy green vegetable has a compound that relaxes the smooth muscle lining in blood vessels, reducing blood pressure. Celery is also a good source of vitamins and minerals, including vitamin C, potassium, calcium and magnesium that help reduce blood pressure. According to a study reported in The New York Times, people who ate four ribs of celery a day lowered their blood pressure by 12 to 14 percent compared with those who did not eat celery.The seed also can be used   to lower blood pressure. Celery is a diuretic, which may help explain its effect on blood pressure.

French Lavender

The beautiful, perfume-like scent of lavender is not the only useful aspect of the plant. Oil of lavender has long been used as a perfume ingredient and also to induce relaxation. The herb may also lower the blood pressure. Although not many people think of using lavender as a culinary herb, the floweris used in baked foods and the leaves can be used in the same way one would use rosemary.

Cat's Claw

Cat's Claw (Uncaria tomentosa) is a woody climbing vine found in South and Central America, with its most notable use being in the Amazon rainforest. It is named after the thorns on the plant which are hooked, much like cats claws. It has been used as a traditional remedy in its native habitat for a long time for hypertension as well as neurological health problems.. It does so by dilating the blood vessels (known as vasodilation) and therefore lowering the pressure by allowing blood to flow through more readily. It can also act as a mild diuretic, getting rid of unneeded salt and water in the body, which can again reduce hypertension. The tannins and flavonoid are most likely the main constituents that account for the herbs healing actions.

Here it is made into a flavorful decoction that will give you all of its benefits. A decoction is essentially a tea, but is simmered for much longer time as it is made from the woody, tough, fibrous parts of the plant such as roots or (in this case) bark., Make sure its scientific name matches the one above (there are several other plants known as cats claw) . Cats Claw should be avoided by women who are pregnant.

Hibiscus

Cultures across the world have used hibiscus to naturally manage blood pressure, but it wasnot until the past decade that studies were actually conducted that showed there was more to the remedy than just folklore. First, hibiscus acts as a diuretic, which draws sodium from the bloodstream, thus decreasing the pressure on the arterial walls. Even more interesting is how it can mimic angiotensin converting enzyme (ACE) inhibitors. ACE inhibitors are a common group of pharmaceutical drugs used to treat high blood pressure. They work by hampering the

angiotensin-converting enzyme, which plays a crucial role in the renin-angiotensin system- a hormone system that regulates blood pressure and fluid balance. As a result of this inhibition, blood vessels relax and blood volume is lowered, decreasing blood pressure.

To lower blood pressure, health professionals with the University of Michigan Health System recommend infusing 1 cup of water with 1 to 2 teaspoons of dried hibiscus flowers. You can consume up to three cups of hibiscus tea daily. Alternatively, drinking one 500 milliliters serving of hibiscus tea each day before breakfast may also help to lower your blood pressure levels
.

Hawthor n

Hawthorn is a staple herb when it comes to heart health as it is rich in flavonoids, Flavonoids are touted as having many benefit for various forms of heart disease. This includes palpitations, improve the function of capillaries, regulate, glucose metabolism and, of course, reduce arterial blood pressure and the risk of hypertension. There are several different mechanical actions that flavonoids can take on the blood, but pertaining to hypertension the most important may be the widening of the blood vessels, which ultimately reduces the pressure of the blood. You can enjoy hawthorn in the form of a tea .

Garlic and Onion

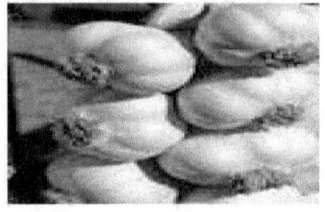 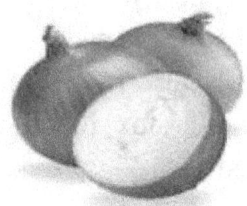

Garlic
Onion
They have both proven to be very effective in reducing blood pressure and blood lipids. Garlic can reduce Systolic pressure by 20 -30 mmHg, and the Diastolic by 10 -20 . Garlic helps to detoxify the body. It is said to stimulate the lymphatic system to throw off waste materials. This powerful natural detoxifier helps to strengthen the blood vessels, providing protection against pollutants and heavy metal toxicity. It also works to cleanse the kidneys and increase urine flow. It reduces the tendency of the blood to clot, thereby increasing circulation and reducing blood pressure and the risk of arteriosclerosis
,stroke and heart attacks. Moreover, Garlic also helps to dilate peripheral blood vessels, thus also helping to balance blood pressure levels. It is also said to play a role in helping to reduce the risk of pre-eclampsia and its complications.

It has anti-inflammatory and antiviral properties that can fight coronary heart disease by unplugging arteries. The gas that garlic produces in the stomach relaxes the arteries and lowers blood pressure. Eating one garlicclove a day can significantly reduce blood pressure within as little as three months. One can also use garlic powder in preparing recipes or take a garlic supplement.

Ginkgo Biloba (Maiden hair, Fossil Tree):

Ginkgo Biloba is one of the oldest living tree species. It is the world's most used natural treatment for memory loss and degenerative diseases of the brain and the central nervous system. It increases the circulation of blood and oxygen to all parts of the body. It has an effect on the entire circulatory system by relaxing the vessels. Its capacity to increase blood flow to the brain helps to prevent strokes, cerebral arteriosclerosis and other diseases of the peripheral circulation. It strengthens micro-circulation in the capillary beds thereby increasing oxygen levels. It also has a significant effect on reducing platelet aggregation. The herb is an effective over-all tonic.

It is a Chinese herb which is available in form of food supplement.

Moring a

The important nutrients needed by a person suffering from high blood pressure are Calcium, Magnesium, Potassium, Zinc, and Vitamin E. Moringa contains these entire nutrient in it. Moringa contains Vitamin C helps support the body's production of nitric oxide, which is critical to normal

47

functioning of blood vessels. The better your blood vessels work, the lower your risk of hypertension. Moringa also contains magnesium along with Zinc and Vitamin E which takes part in decreasing the blood pressure along with other nutrients

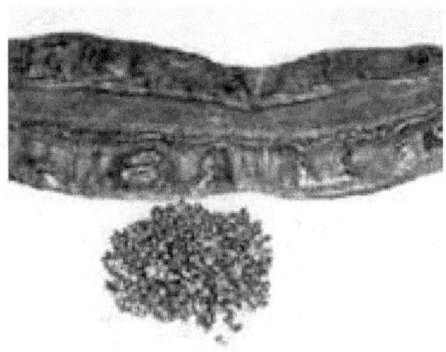

Tetrapleuratetrapte ra

Tetrapleuratetraptera belongs to the mimosaceae family. It is referred locally to as Aridan in Yoruba and Oshosho in Ibo

Researchers have found that regular intake of the fruit and bark extracts of this   local spice, could prevent the development of hypertension and its complications.

It has also   been used in folk medicine in the treatment of hypertensive disorders, inflammation and several women's diseases such as breast and uterus cancers, in diabetics and cardiovascular treatment.

This plant is also frequently used in Tropical African traditional medicine for the management and/or control of other array of human ailments including arthritis , inflammatory conditions, asthma, diabetes mellitus, hypertension and epilepsy

SOME DRINKS THAT LOWER BLOOD PRESSURE

Some drinks can contribute to a drop in blood pressure, especially in combination with a healthy diet and regular exercise.

Coconut Water

Coconut water is found inside the shell of green, unripe coconuts that retains its natural benefits in organic and raw form.

Coconut water is filled with potassium and magnesium electrolytes, which are good for the heart muscle.Coconut water lowers blood pressure by acting as a potassium sparing diuretic. This removes the excess water from the body, while retaining vital potassium.Coconut water is best when it is organic and bottled in its raw form.Drink 8 ounces of organic coconut water, 1-3 times a day. The effects are weight based, so if you are on the heavier side, drink more coconut water (3 times a day).

Low-fat milk

Calcium deficiencies have long been linked to high

blood

pressure, and high calcium intake helps lower high blood pressure. It is important to choose the right type of milk for the best results, though. Low-fat milk is richer in calcium than full- fat milk, and the modest amount of fat actually helps in absorbing the calcium more easily. As part of a daily regimen, three servings of low-fat milk and other low-fat dairy products has been shown to help reduce systolic blood pressure.

Beet juice

Beets are a good source of potassium -- and a good source of folate, both of which are important in regulating blood pressure. Beets contain nitrate, which is converted into nitrites once ingested. Nitrites relax smooth muscle tissue and increase blood flow. Finally, beets support healthy blood vessel function and battle homocysteine, which can damage blood vessels.

Research suggests that one to two cups of beet juice daily can lower blood pressure immediately (within an hour of consumption) and significantly. An English study found beet juice to be as effective as nitrate tablets in treating hypertension.

Pomegranate juice

ACE is an enzyme that raises blood pressure by creating a protein called angiotensin II, which causes your blood vessels to constrict. Pomegranate juice acts as a natural ACE inhibitor, similar to the class of medications prescribed to treat hypertension and heart failure. In one case, pomegranate juice reduced ACE by 36 percent and lowered systolic blood pressure, too. It also had been shown in a handful of recent studies to significantly reduced (up to 30 percent) arterial plaque and increased blood flow to the heart.

Sipping suggestion: Nutrition guru Jonny Bowden recommends drinking six ounces of unsweetened pomegranate juice every day. Too tart? Have two three-ounce servings cut with water or sparkling mineral water.

Cranberry
juice
How it works: Cranberries and cranberry juice have powerful anti-inflammatory and antioxidant properties that help prevent and reduce damage inside the blood vessels, thereby preventing an undesirable increase in blood pressure. In addition, cranberry juice may help reduce blood pressure by dilating blood vessels and increasing blood flow. Finally, cranberries are an excellent source of blood-pressure-lowering vitamin C.

Sipping suggestion: There's no standard recommendation for the amount of cranberry juice to drink as part of a daily regimen, but be sure to go for the unsweetened variety that's
100-percent cranberry juice. At 60 calories per one-cup serving, you can have two servings and still get fewer calories than you'd get with the sweetened stuff, which averages about 130 calories per cup.

Water

How it works: Drinking adequate amounts of water is, quite simply, one of the healthiest, cheapest, and most effective ways that you can help lower your blood pressure. Chronic dehydration causes blood vessels to constrict, which helps the body conserve water by reducing water loss through perspiration, urination, and respiration. Unfortunately, constricted blood vessels require your heart to work harder, resulting in a spike in blood pressure.

Herb/ Green tea

Herb teas such as Chamomile, Fennel, Mistletoe [on Cola nut and citrus family] and Rose Mary are veritable remedy for high blood pressure. The mistletoe leaves should be dried under room temperature and taken as tea by steeping one tea spoon in a cup of hot water for about ten minutes before straining and drinking. Do this twice , morning and evening daily.

Scientific studies point to green tea as a food that can help reverse some of the risk factors associated with heart disease, including high blood pressure and abnormal blood clotting. Much of the research on green tea has been conducted in Japan, where men and women drink a high daily intake of green tea, and also have one of the lowest incidences of heart disease in the world

Sipping suggestion:
For a more personalized approach, divide your body weight in two. That figure -- in ounces -- is minimum water you should aim to drink per day. For example, a 150-pound person should shoot for at least 75 ounces daily

Apple cider vinegar: Vinegar alkalizes the body and lowers blood pressure.

First thing in the morning, when the stomach is empty, drink 8 ounces of warm water mixed with 1 table spoon of apple cider vinegar and 1 tsp honey regularly. The honey ensures regularity of bowel movement, which is helpful since constipation may aggravate high blood pressure

Cocoa beverage : It had been discovered that the daily intake of hot cocoa will decrease the risks of elevated blood pressure and cardiovascular failure. It also improves the over-all function of the cells lining the blood vessels and works to stimulate the body's production of nitric oxide. Hot cocoa actually thins the blood thereby allowing an increase of blood flow to the heart, brain and other pertinent organs. The use of cocoa is borrowed from the citizens of central America, especially the Kuna Indians living on Coastal island of Panama.

The Kuna Indians are free from high blood pressure which can be attributed to their regular consumption of hot cocoa which not only lower the blood pressure but also improves the over-all functions of the cells lining the blood vessels.

It also works to stimulate the body production of nitric oxide.

The hot cocoa actually thins the blood allowing an increase

in
blood flow to the heart, the brain and other parts of the body. Harvard researchers also submit that hot cocoa can also be used to treat blocked arteries, congested heart failure, stroke and other ailments.

FRUITS AND VEGETABLE FOR LOWERING BLOOD PRESSURE
Eating a balanced array of fresh wholesome fruits and vegetables of all color everyday is of great benefits for blood pressure

Broccol
i
Sulforaphane Glucosinolate (SGS), a naturally-occurring compound found in broccoli helps in reducing high blood pressure as well as cardiovascular disease and stroke risk.

Cabbag
e
Cabbage is high in a chemical compound called glutamic acid, which helps in reducing blood pressure. Glutamic acid is the most common amino acid and accounts for almost a

quarter of vegetable protein and nearly a fifth of animal protein.

Mistletoe *(Viscum album)*

Mistletoe is a hemi-parasitic plant in the sandalwood family. Aqueous extracts of its leaves display blood pressure lowering effects in animal studies. Mistletoe on Cola nut and citrus trees are effective.

Wild African black plum *(Vitexdoniana)*

An extract from this flowering plant in the mint family has significantly lowered blood pressure in animal studies.

African corkwood tree (Musangacecropioides)

Native to Africa, this straight-stemmed evergreen tree has been studied for its effects on lowering blood pressure.

Basil *(Ocimumbasilicum)*

This South East Asian culinary herb exhibits antihypertensive effects through its chemical compound, eugenol. Also found in spices such as cinnamon, nutmeg, and clove, eugenol works by blocking calcium channels.

Black mangrove *(Lumnitzeraracemosa)*

Amongst the mangrove plants, the black mangrove is the most salt tolerant species. An aqueous acetone extract of this small tree has been shown to display antihypertensive activity.

River lily *(Crinum*

glaucum)

An aqueous extract of this West Nigerian plant has been shown to reduce both systolic and diastolic blood pressures.

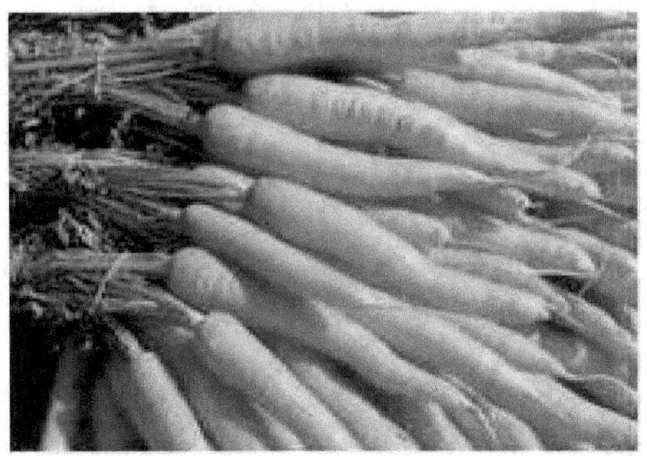

Carrot

Carrot cleans up the arteries. Carrot juice is high in beta-carotene, which studies show can reduce the risk of heart disease, which may lead to high blood pressure. The juice helps to maintain normal blood pressure by regulating heart and kidney measure of carrot and celery juices in water be taken at least once daily.

Celery
Oriental medicine practitioners have long used celery for reducing high blood pressure. There is some experimental evidence which shows that celery is useful for this. A research has shown that eating as few as four celery stalks a day canreduce high blood pressure. However, celery contains sodium and other compounds that may have side effects when consumed in large amounts.

Cucumber:

As a natural diuretic, cucumber will help hydrate and lower the pressure in the arteries.
Eat 2 fresh cucumbers every day for 2 weeks .

Grape fruit:

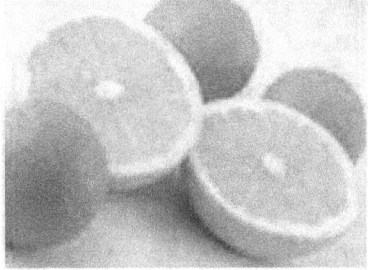

The vitamin P content in grape fruit is very helpful in toning up the arteries and lowering the blood pressure

Water melon

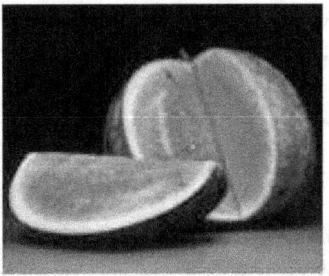

Water lemon is particularly a multivitamin unto itself. It contains Vitamins A, B6 and C. It also contains Beta carotene and Lycopene which is an anti-oxidant that protects the human heart. The deep red variety of water melon displaces tomato as the Lycopene king.

Water melon both relaxes and increases the diameter of the arteries. Is believed to have Viagra –like effect on the body blood vessel, thus helping to lower the high blood pressure . It is said to be a major player in the diet of the Mediterranean countries which had protected the people of the region against heart disease.

Every morning, be faithful to watermelon. It contains an organic compound called citrulline, an a-amino acid, which when ingested, the body converts citrulline to the amino acid L-arginine, which is a precursor to nitric oxide.. Nitric oxide affects various cells and systems in the body that regulates, among other things, how hard your blood gets pumped through your entire body-also known as vascular systematic resistance. It will widen blood vessels, which lowers vascular resistance, which

Please note that water melon should not be eaten along with other fruits but alone ,either about thirty minutes before or after for full benefit.

Fresh pawpaw

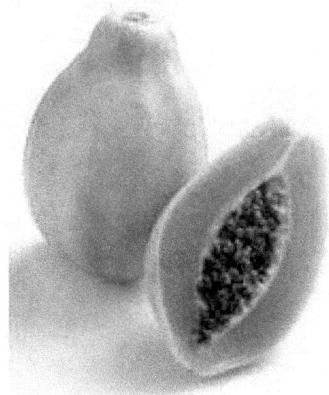

The liberal amount of potassium in pawpaw helps in checking blood pressure and improving mental alertness .It also provides protection against heart disease because the nutrients in papaya prevents the oxidation of cholesterol which when becomes oxidized is able to stick to and build up in the artery walls to form dangerous plaques.Take fresh pawpaw daily on an empty stomach regularly to relieve hypertension.

Banana s

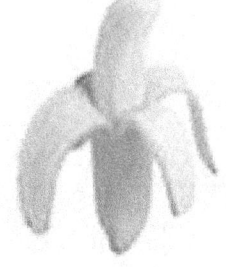

Bananas have a high content of potassium, which is known to lower blood pressure and reduce the risk of stroke. Bananas are also low in sodium, which is important for people with high blood pressure to avoid. Just one banana a day can provide a dose of potassium, helping to reduce blood pressure and fend off various cardiovascular diseases. Along with bananas, you can also eat other fruits such as apples, plums, pears, pomegranate, and mangoes. It is also rich in powerful antioxidants, Vitamins C and A and element Zinc. It also helps in boosting the body immune system.

Avocados
Pear

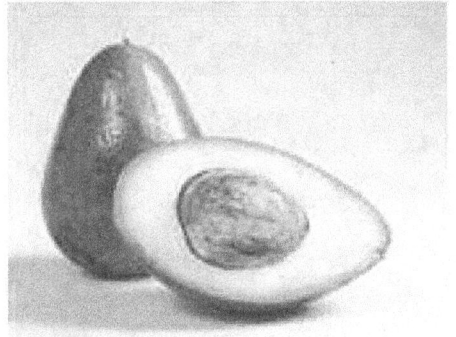

Avocados contain Folate , Potassium, mono-saturated fats and are very high in fiber which is known to help prevent high blood pressure, heart disease and certain types of cancer. It contains more Potassium than banana; Potassium is beneficial to the body by lowering the risk of high blood pressure, heart attack and cancer. The mono-saturated fats has been found to improve fat levels in the body and thereby help control diabetes. In addition the mono-saturated fats ,the oleic acid found in avocados can reduces cholesterol levels. They also contain potassium and folate, which both essential for heart health. The seed is also effective in curing high blood pressure

in two ways ; the first is by boiling about ten seeds in about five litres of water till they become very soft and straining and sieving off the water. The dosage is one glass each in the morning and evening. The second method is by cutting the seeds in pieces and drying under room temperature before grinding into powder. The dosage is by steeping one tea-spoon in a cup of hot water for ten minutes andallowing to cool before drinking. This should be repeated twice daily.

Cayenne   /Chili Pepper

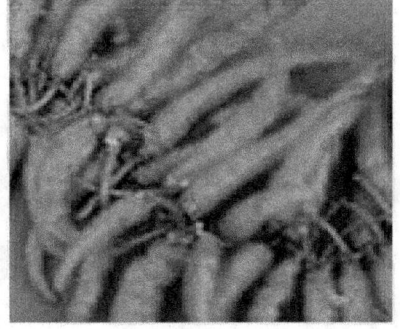

Cayenne is one of the best known folk remedies for high blood pressure. As a cardiovascular stimulant, cayenne is believed to help strengthen the heart, regulate the blood pressure, lower blood lipids ,reduce the peripheral resistance in the capillary beds and dilate the blood vessel diameter . It is said to improve blood circulation and is thought to normalize both high and low blood pressure .It apparently increases heart action without increasing the blood pressure.   Cayenne reportedly, significantly lowers serum cholesterol and triglycerides. It is also said to speed up the metabolism of fat and may reduce weight gain due to high fat diet by increasing the liver enzymes accountable for fat metabolism.

Dark chocolate

Dark chocolate is not only tasty, but it also good for our health. A recent study found that eating a small amounts of dark chocolate every day lowered the systolic blood pressure by 2.9mm Hg and diastolic by 1.9mm Hg. The key ingredient of dark chocolate is flavanols that is present in cocoa. Not all chocolate will do, but a good quality dark chocolate that has 60 to 70 percent of cocoa.

Sunflower seeds

Sunflower seeds contain phytosterols, which can reduce cholesterol levels , a well-known contributor to high blood pressure because it can cause blockage of blood vessels. However, make sure that you are using fresh sunflower seeds.

Sesame (Sesamumindicum)

Sesame is one of the oldest oil-seed crops known. In patients with hypertension, consumption of sesame oil has been shown to reduce oxidative stress and increase endogenous antioxidant production. Sesamin, a lignan found in sesame oil, may be useful as a preventative for hypertension

VITAMINS AND MINERALS FOR LOWERING BLOOD PRESSURE

Vitamins
:
Eat vitamin-rich foods. A daily consumption of multivitamins ensures you are eating right.

Vitamin C: The less this vitamin, in the blood, the higher the blood pressure in hypertension patient.
Bioflanoids; It enhances vitamin C effect. It is available in fruits and vegetables.
Vitamin E:Evidence shows that it also magnifies vitamin C
blood pressure –lowering effect.

Potassium is essential: Those with high blood pressure are often found to be Potassium- deficient . Potassium deficiency causes the cells to take up sodium which in turn causes the blood pressure to rise. Tell-tale sign of low potassium include irregular heart beats slower reflexes among others.

Potassium-associated blood pressure reduction significantly lowers the risk of stroke, coronary heart disease, and other cardiovascular events. Taking of 4.7 grams a day of potassium, may lead to a decrease of up to 15% risk of

stroke and up to
11% in risk of heart attack

This crucial mineral is found in many fruits and vegetables, bananas, potatoes ,diary foods and fish.

Magnesium: It is also a crucial mineral ,it is present in leafy greens, legumes and whole grains

Honey: Honey is known to be a Heart re-activator or Cardiac cleanser. Blend of honey and garlic cures hypertension and some infectious diseases in blood.

Similarly a regular use of a mixture of 5mls each of onion and honey, taken twice daily, cures pretension.
A blend of ginger and garlic with honey enhances the heart functions.
.

Calcium: People who take Potassium and Calcium – rich diets have low incidence of high blood pressure. These two essential nutrients help the body to get rid of excess sodium and are involved in important functions which control the working of the vascular system.Calcium is important for healthy blood pressure because it helps blood vessels tighten and relax when they need to.

It is also crucial for healthy bones and the release of hormones and enzymes we need for most body functions. We consume it naturally in dairy products, yogurt and cheese (the skim or low fat varieties which are richer in calcium are recommended) ,fish with bones (such as canned salmon and sardines), and dark, leafy greens.

Calcium could prevent the hypertensive disorders known as "preeclampsia" and "eclampsia" In pregnant women . In studies where some women were given at least one gram of calcium daily during their pregnancy, the risk of pre-eclampsia and preterm birth were reduced by 50%.

Calcium obtained naturally from food is more effective than supplements. It should also be noted that Calcium works more effectively in conjunction with Magnesium.

Omega-3 and Omega 6 :

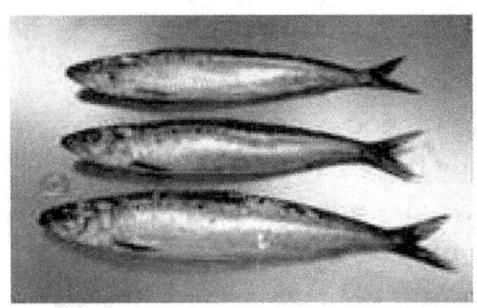

Mackerel

These fatty acids are found in fish such as salmon, Mackerel, Sardine and Herring. They are also found in flax seed oil and Primrose oil. Of all animal products, fish is the healthiest, owing to its high protein and low fat content. The omega-3 fatty acids in fish, along with other nutrients, protect blood vessels from plaque, reduce inflammation, and prevent high blood pressure.

The fish oil lower blood pressure, controls cholesterol, makes the arteries more flexible and helps in keeping blood platelets from clotting together along the artery walls. This keeps the passages open and the blood flowing through freely so there is less pressure on the arteries. However, fish with high mercury content such as Tuna which may increase the blood pressure should be avoided

COQ10:

Hypertensive patients are often found to be deficient in coenzyme Q10 usually called COQ10 . It is also known as Ubiquinone meaning the ubiquitous quinine.

Coenzyme Q10 has been shown to be beneficial for treating heart disease, atherosclerosis and hypertension and various other ailments.

It is essentially a vitamin or a vitamin-like substance ,which like vitamins are found in foods and sometimes synthesized in the body. It is fat-soluble and present in all cells of the body where it serves as a coenzyme and also functions as an antioxidant.

It is naturally present in small amounts in a wide variety of foods but is particularly high in organ meats such as heart, liver and kidney as well as in beef, soy oil , sardines, mackerel and peanuts. Given all the nutrients and vitamins that it needs, the body will manufacture its own supply of

COQ10.

It's usually best to get calcium, magnesium, and potassium from food. Are you getting enough?

Potassiu
m

Normal body levels of potassium are important for muscle function, including relaxing the walls of the blood vessels. This lowers blood pressure and protects against muscle cramping. Normal potassium levels also are important for the conduction of electrical signals in the nervous system and in the heart. This protects against an irregular heartbeat.

Potassium is found naturally in many foods, such as prunes, apricots, sweet potatoes, and lima beans. Food may not be enough to keep up your potassium levels if you take a diuretic for high blood pressure. This causes potassium to leave your body through in the urine, thereby lowering your body's potassium levels.

Magnesiu
m

Magnesium helps regulate hundreds of body systems, including blood pressure, blood sugar, and muscle and nerve function. We need magnesium to help blood vessels relax, and for energy production, bone development, and transporting calcium and potassium. Just like potassium, too much magnesium can be lost in urine due to diuretic use, leading to low magnesium levels.

It is best to get the mineral from food, especially dark, leafy green vegetables, unrefined grains, and legumes..

Too much magnesium from a supplement or from magnesium- containing drugs such as laxatives may cause diarrhea. There are no known adverse affects of magnesium intake from food.

SOME 42 WAYS TO PREVENT OR LOWER BLOOD PRESSURE

DASH -
DASH is the acronym for Dietary Approach to Stop Hypertension

Dietary Approaches to Stop Hypertension (DASH) is an eating plan to lower or control high blood pressure.

It is an over-all eating plan that focuses on what people should eat rather than what not to eat. It is rich in fruits, vegetables, grains, fiber, complex carbohydrates and low – fat dairy products ; it is low in fat, saturated fat, cholesterol and sodium and higher in Potassium, Magnesium and Calcium. A healthy eating plan can both reduce the risk of developing high blood pressure and lower an already high blood pressure.

It is a flexible and balanced eating plan that helps creates a heart- healthy eating style for life and requires no special foods but instead provides daily and weekly nutritional goals. This plan recommends:

Eating vegetables, fruits, and whole grains including fat-free or low-fat dairy products, fish, poultry, beans, nuts, and vegetable ns, fish, poultry and nuts. It offers limited portions of red meats, sweets and sugary beverages.Oils limiting foods that are high in saturated fat, such as fatty meats, full-fat dairy products, and tropical oils such as palm kernel, and palm oils . It also limits sugar-sweetened beverages and sweets

Life-style change

Lifestyle plays an important role in treating   high blood pressure   and adopting a good life style will go a long way to reduce high blood pressure .

Listed   below are some positive and helpful life-style:

Fight stress:

Stress or anxiety can temporarily increase blood pressure. It is good   to take some time to think about what may be causing one   to feel stressed, such as work, family, finances or illness. Once this is known , consider how you can eliminate or reduce the   stress. Also adopt healthy habits to fight stress because this can protect one from the harmful effects .

Daily dose of friendship; This is a great medicine ,call or chat with friends and those around you to share your feeling, hopes and joy.

regular

Daily

activities, Exercise:

Along with diet, exercise should really be number one on this list. Nothing can replace what exercise does for the body, and in a society where we are becoming increasingly sedentary, it can take a bit more effort to get out and get moving-but it's worth it, especially if you have high blood pressure. The heart is a muscle, and it will grow stronger with exercise. It becomes easier to pump blood and takes less effort, keeping your heart in better condition and lowering how much force it exerts on the arteries, thus lowering blood pressure. Exercise is, in many cases, all that one needs to get blood pressure back on track. The top number in a blood pressure reading indicates systolic blood pressure, which is created by the heart pumping blood away from it. Exercise can lower this reading by an average of 4 to 9 millimeters of mercury (a unit of pressure), which is easily as much as some prescription blood pressure medications. A pleasant side effect of exercise is weight loss, which also does your heart and arteries a great favor. regular physical activity relieves mental and physical tension. Physically active people have lower risk of depression and loss of mental functioning.

Try not to worry or be anxious: Accept things you cannot

change and avoid unnecessary worries or care. The world will not end if your lawn is not mowed-you may need to do this, but it may not be necessarily now. Cast all your care and worries upon the Lord ,for He careth for you. " ..Be anxious for nothing ,but in prayer and supplication with thanksgiving let your request be made known unto God..." {I Peter 5: 7 ; Philippians 4:6}

✏️ **Learn to laugh:** Laughter makes you feel good and relieved. Do not shy or be afraid to laugh out loud at a joke or a funny movie a comic strip or whenever occasions call for it , even when alone.

✏️ **Give up the bad habits:** Avoid smoking, alcohol ,or caffeine All these can increase stress. So quit them now.

✏️ **Slow down:** Learn to "pace" instead of "race". Always plan ahead and allow enough time to get the most important things done. Always spread out activities and projects; avoid lumping up. Take one day at a time.

✏️ **Get organized:** Always wake up in time so as to be able to start the day without rushing. You may adopt the use of a check - list, a what-to-do list, to help you focus on your important tasks. Always approach tasks ,one step at a time. Try as much as possible to simplify and un-clutter your life.

✏️ **Always get enough sleep:** In stead of skimping on sleep to add hours to your day get more in order to add years to your life. According to an expert " Sleep is one of the most important functions that the body uses to regulate and heal the cells." Try to get six to eight hours of sleep each night. Physical activities also may improve the quality of sleep.

- Say "No" to Projects /activities that will not fit into your time schedule, or that will compromise your mental health.

- Learn to delegate tasks to capable hands, but remember that "Delegation is no Relegation".

- Pay adequate attention to time :Allow sufficient time to do things and to attend to events or programmes punctually.

- Separate worries from concerns. If a situation is a concern, find out what God would have you do and let go of anxiety. If you cannot do any thing about a situation, forget about it .Remember   that no one "......by taking thought   can add one cubit unto his stature "- Matthew 6:27

- Live within your budget.

- Like a good IT. Expert, always keep   back-ups : For your computer files , keep your extra car   key handy and Your house extra keys in an easily accessible place .

- Eat right and thereby live well.

- Relax your mind when caught up in the traffic "Hold-up" or "Go –slow" by listening to good music .

Having problems? Nip such problems in the bud by talking instantly to God on the spot .Remember to " Pray incessantly" - I Thess.5: 17. Also remember that the shortest bridge between despair and hope is a short breath of prayer such as " Jesus cover me with Your Blood " or Jesus ! "The Name of the Lord is a Strong Tower......" Prov.18:10.

Always exercise a forgiving spirit, habouring no malice or
ill-feeling. Always like Apostle Paul in Acts 4 :16- ".....have a conscience free of offence towards God and towards men."

Learn talk less and listen more. Remember that a minute of silence/thought is worth more than an hour of talk.

Read check food labels. If possible, choose low-sodium alternatives of the foods and beverages you normally buy. Eat fewer processed foods. Potato chips, frozen dinners, bacon and processed lunch meats are high in sodium.

Shaff salt: Avoid all sodium-rich food like the fast foods and snacks. It is a known fact that sodium is hidden in packaged foods even in higher quantities than people are aware of. It is also interesting to note that eating natural and unprocessed fruits ,vegetables, meat and fish

provides all the sodium the body
needs.

There is however no reason why avoiding or eating less salt or sodium should make food less delicious because certain herbs and spices can make food spicy without salt and sodium.

High blood pressure sufferer who keep a low-salt diet can expect an average systolic blood pressure reduction of 4.0-

6.0 mmHg and a diastolic blood pressure reduction of 2.0-

3.0 mmHg.

FOOD LABELS

Pay very close attention to food labels on processed foods because they account for most of the salt and sodium consumed. Processed food high in salt include regular canned vegetables and soups, frozen dinners, instant , ready- to -eat cereals , salty chips and snacks.

Sodium reduction drops blood pressure by about 3.5%

for those with high blood
pressure.

Listed below are some suggested spices and herbs as good alternatives to table salt:

- Basil -driedin- door and ground into powder.
- Chili powder-dried and powdered chili pepper
- Ginger
-

-      ”   ”   ”
Nutmeg-   ”   ”   ”
Parley -   ”   ”   ”
Rosemary ”   ”   ”

- Thyme-   "   "   "   "
- Garlic   "   "   "   "

- **Fiber:** Eat lots of vegetables and whole grains. The healthiest diet is a high fiber diet that contains whole grains, fruits, vegetables and lean meats. Fiber is critical for flushing the body of toxins cholesterol and plague build-up.

- **Go for oats:** When eaten daily, oats lower hypertension.
Oats and oat bran contain a specific type of fiber known as beta-glucan which have been shown to reduce blood pressure and cholesterol levels. Eating a serving of oats at least 6 times each week is an especially good idea for postmenopausal women with high cholesterol, high blood pressure or other signs of cardiovascular disease.

- **Defeat Diabetes:** Diabetics should control their condition in order to reduce the risk of hypertension.

- **Watch weight :** Ensure that your BMI is between 18.5 and 24.9.Being overweight or obese increases the risk of developing high blood pressure. In fact the blood pressure rises as the weight increases, losing even 10 pounds can lower the blood pressure Losing weight has the biggest effect on those who are overweight and hypertensive. Risk factors are increased when added weight is in the abdominal area of the body. There is a significant risk factor for developing high blood pressure for obese people,

The two key measures used to determine the condition of overweight and obesity are the Body Mass Index and The waist circumference. A waist measurement of more than 35 inches for women and more than 40 for men is considered high. However it is important to note that weight loss should be done slowly as stated earlier.

2- Whole –Grain :Eating more whole-grain foods on a regular basis may help reduce your chance of developing high blood pressure (hypertension).

Whole grains are grains that include the entire grain kernel
- their bran and germ had not been removed by refining. Whole-grain foods are a rich source of healthy nutrients, including fiber, potassium, magnesium and foliate. Eating more whole-grain foods offers many health benefits that can work together to help reduce the risk of high blood pressure by aiding in weight control, since whole-grain foods can make one feels full longer .

3- Increasing your intake of potassium, which is linked
to

lower blood pressure

Decreasing your risk of insulin resistance

Reducing damage to your blood vessels.

If you already have high blood pressure, eating more whole- grain foods might help lower your blood pressure and possibly reduce your need for blood pressure medication. According to the Dietary Guidelines for Americans, as part of an overall healthy diet, adults should eat at least 85 grams of whole-grain foods a day - about 3 ounces, or the equivalent of three slices of whole-wheat bread.

The Three Bs: consuming diet rich in vitamins B1, B6 and B12 reduce the risk of arteries clotting. There are food supplements having them in combination.

Hydrotherapy;

A good proactive approach is to drink water regularly. This is a good way to cleanse and refresh every part of the body, even the blood vessels. Many of the drugs usually prescribed to lower blood pressure are basically diuretics and water is a natural diuretic. Drink eight to ten glasses daily to flush out excess salt and toxins that may be in the blood stream. Water is a good replacement for some drinks containing caffeine which temporarily raises the blood pressure.

Hot foot or Leg bath for 10-15 minutes and a Hot compress over the heart are other water treatments that have been proved beneficial for treating high blood pressure.

MORE FOODS TO AVOID

The following foods which tend to aggravate hypertension should be strictly avoided:
Licorice, Anise seed, St. John's wort , Capsaicin, Ginseng, Parsley, Blue cohosh, Vervain , Bayberry and Chasteberry.

It is however important to note that foods that are helpful for lowering blood pressure , Hypertension , should be avoided as soon as the blood pressure becomes normal so that it does not become Hypotension , Low blood pressure. Such herbs include Garlic, Hawthorn, Olive leaf, Onion, Hibiscus, Indian snakeroot, European mistletoe, Reishi and mushrooms .

- **FoFgo;** Choose white fish and skinless chicken and turkey. Avoid cheese, bacon and red meat. Also toss the trans fats which are even of greater risk than the saturated fats.

- **Coffee** : Caffeine in coffee can cause a temporary but sharp rise in blood pressure. Exactly what causes this spike in blood pressure is uncertain but someresearchers have suggested that caffeine narrows blood vessels by blocking the effects of adenosine, a hormone that helps keep them widened. Caffeine may also stimulate the adrenal gland to release more cortisol and adrenaline, which causes   the blood pressure to increase.

Refined Sugar:

Limit   intake of sugar and saturated fats as they can increase inflammation and harden the arteries, contributing to hypertension

The average person consumes nearly 240 pounds of sugar per year. Most of the excess sugar ends up being stored as fat in your body, resulting in weight gain and elevating heart disease and cancer risk. Sugar makes blood pressure rise, especially in people who are overweight.

Honey contains vitamins and minerals that are lacking in refined table sugar, making it much healthier for you. Instead of refined sweets, go for the natural delicious flavors of fresh fruit and berries.

Alcohol:

Researches   have seen an association between the consumption of alcohol and rise in blood pressure . Among the risk factors for hypertension alcohol is second only to obesity in its   observed contribution to the prevalence of hypertension in men . Several studies had also found that drinking excessive amounts of alcohol can raise blood pressure to unhealthy levels. Also, it should be kept   in mind that alcohol contains calories and may contribute to unwanted weight gain- a risk factor for high blood pressure. Worse still, alcohol can interfere with the effectiveness and increase the side effects of some blood pressure medications.

Smoking:
Avoid smoking like a plague because all forms of tobacco raise blood pressure. Smoking is a major cause of cardiovascular disease, including heart attacks ,strokes and peripheral artery disease. It damages blood vessels.

You should also avoid second-hand smoke; inhaling smoke from others also puts one at risk of health problems, including high blood pressure and heart disease.

Refine d foods:
Shun the salty, sugary, preserved ,fried and fatty foods.

Soda: Soft drinks and synthetic fruit juice can deplete
potassium in the body.

Caffeine: Avoiding the consumption of high caffeine , sodium and excessive sugar.
Some life style factors contributing to high blood pressure which shoul be avoided are smoking, stress levels , sedentary work, and alcohol consumption .

Chapter Six

GLOSSARY- DEFINITIONS OF SOME CIRCULATORY TERMS USED IN THIS BOOK

Anemia - Insufficient red cells or hemoglobin in the blood

Artery - Large blood vessel that carry oxygenated blood away from the heart to the other parts of the body.

Arteriosclerosis - The thickening and hardening of the arteries due to the build-up of calcium deposits on the internal artery walls.

Atherosclerosis - Accumulation of plaques, build-up of fatty substances on the internal walls of the arteries.

Antimutagenic - capable of reducing the frequency of mutation.

Antitumorigenic- Serving to counteract the the

formation of tumors.

Blood - Red fluid that carries oxygen and nutrients to the cells and takes away carbon dioxide and waste.

Blood Lipids - blood fats

Capillary - Smallest part of the blood vessel that distribute the nutrients and oxygen to the body tissues and remove deoxygenated blood and waste..

Cardiac - elating to the heart.

Cardiovascular - Relating to the heart and the circulatory system.

Cholesterol - Fatty molecules in the blood produced by the liver. Good cholesterol is called HDL(high-density lipoprotein). It is linked to a reducd risk of \hear and blood vessel disease while bad one is called LDL (Low density lipoprotein)and is linked to an increase risk of cardiovascular disease , including coronary artery disease.

Coronary disease -   Heart problem due to lack of sufficient flow of blood.

Diastolic blood pressure - The lowest blood pressure between heart beats.

Diuretic - An agent that increases the flow of urine.

Endocrine - Hormones in the blood stream.

Hemoglobin - Oxygen-carrying red blood

cell. **Hemorrhage** - Bleeding

Hemostasis - Clotting **Hypertension** -

High blood pressure. **Hypotension** - Low

blood pressure. **Hypoxemia** - Low level of

blood in the body. **Macrocytes** -

Abnormally large blood cells

Magnesium - Blood salt.
Microcytes - Abnormally small blood cells

Platelet - or Thrombocytes are
irregularly-

shaped colourless bodies present in the blood.Their sticky surface let them along with other substances form clots, they play a fundamental role in hemostasis leading to formation of blood clot;if too low causes excessive bleeding and on the other hand if too high causes blood and result in the obstruction of the blood vessels.

CHAPTER SEVEN

NIGERIAN NATIVE NAMES OF SOME COMMON HERBS AND SPICES

Tabulated below are the Nigerian native names of some common herbs and spices, including those mentioned in this book.

Item nos	English/Botanical name	Hausa	Igbo	Yoruba
	Miracle fruit			Agbayun
	Alligator pepper			Atare
	Bitter leave	Shiwaka	Olubgbu	Ewuro
	Garlic	Tafarnuuwa	Ayo	Ayu
	Ginger	Cittar	Jinja	Atale
	Sweet basil		Nchanwun	Efinrin
	Clove			Kannafuru
	Thorny pig weed			Teteelegun
	Cayenne pepper			Shombo
	Turmeric			Atale pupa
	cashew	Kanju	Kausu	Kaju
	Hog plum	Tsadarmasar	Jikara/ogogo	Iyeye
	Sodom apple	Bambambele		Bomubomu
	Star bur	Ewe duba		Dagunro

Goat weed		Agadinwanyii siawo	Imiesu
Tree of life, Fertility tree	Aduruku	Ogilisi	Akoko
Cock's comb	Kalkashn-koorama	Asuuzo	Ogbeakuko
Never die		Odaopue	Abamoda
African cucumber/ Bitter gourd	Daddagu	Aloose, Akbanndene	Ejinrin
Pig nut	Da zugu	Oluluidu	Lapalapa
African wall nut		Ukpa	Asala
Wild mango	Gooronbirii	Ogbono	Oro abeje
Sweet basil	Dandoriya	Nchu-anwu	Efinrinwewe
Avocado pear		Ube oyibo	Pia
Black tamarind	Tsamiyarkurmi	Icheku	Awin
senna		Ogaalu	Asuwonoyinbo
Crab's eyes	Idonzakara	Anya Nnunu	Ojuologbo
Cam wood	Majigi	Ufie,Abosi	Igiosun
Horse eye	Marara	Agbala	Werepe
Aloe vera	Zabo		Ewe etierin
Climbing lily	Gudumarzome	Obaraokpa	Akalamagbo
Henna plant	Lallee	Laali	Laali
Hibiscus		Ireagu	Kekeke
Sorrel	Zoborodo	Okworo-ozo	Isapa pupa
Velvet leaf	Fiyaka	Abakenwo	Jokoje
African oak	Loko	Oji	Iroko
Sand paper	Baure	Anwerenwa	Epin
Plantain	Ayabarturawa	OgedeOyibo	Ogedeagbagba
Guinea corn	Gero	Oka maajali	Poroporo -baba
Chilli pepper	Barkono	Ose	Ata jije
Edible-stemed vine	Da'ddori	Ogbakiikii	Eyun,Ororo

109

INDEX

Caffeine 67

SUFFIXES AND PREFIXES

Cardio	-	heart
Cyte	-	cell
Haem	-	Blood
Thromb	-	Clot, lump
Ethro	-	Red
Leuko	-	White
Vas	-	Vessel/Duct
Hyper	-	Excessive
Hypo	-	Deficient
	-	Penia Deficiency
	-	Emia Condition of blood

BIBILOGRAPH

1. The clinician's handbook of natural medicine-JE Pizzomo,MMurray, H.Joiner-Bey

2. Lycopene and health- Barbara Levine, Ph.D., R.D.

3. High Blood Pressure: A significant problem with herbs being a significant answer- Terry Williad

4   Expert Questions and Answers Eating to control high blood presure-An Interview with Dean Ormish .MD.

5. Eat Right and live well - T.A. Shobukola

6. Great Reading Home- Holistic living

7. Hot cocoa for treating high blood pressure.

8   A new home Remedy to lower High blood pressure-Alvin Hopkinson

9   Nutritional Remedies for common Ailments - T.A.Shobukola.

10. Alcohol Health and Research-World summer 1990

11. The best Natural ways to lower your blood pressure.-

12. Interview Tom   Vento and Frank Mangano .

13 . Nikki Jong,- Caring.com contributing editor

14. The Holy Bible- King James version.

15. The Healthline Editorial Team

16 . Everyday Roots Book

17. John Summerly PreventDisease.com

18. healthimpactnews.com/2014/9-herbs-and-plants-
     that-   will-lower-your-blood-pressure-naturally/
     #sthash.V U9AZ7mC.dpuf

19. Harvard Health Letter

20. DASH -Mayo Clinic Staff

21. Medicinal Plants of Nigeria
     - Nigeria Natural Medicine Development Agency

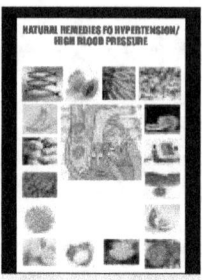

T he book, Natural Remedies for high blood pressure is
another publication in the Nutritional remedies series.
It is a humble attempt at presenting simple and natural
home remedies for the ubiquitous silent killer, which respects
neither age nor race, in a simple and easy to understand
manner.

The Author, Engr. T.A.Shobukola MBA ;MNSE;MNIM. is
a self-developed Advocate for a natural ,non-drug approach
for body ailments by applying the abundant God-given
nutritional remedies for human health.

He is the author of other previous fast - selling publications
among which are "EAT RIGHT AND LIVE WELL" ,
"NUTRITIONAL REMEDIES FOR COMMON AILMENTS" ',
PROSTATE CARE','HEALING HERBS AND SPICES','NATURAL
SOURCES OF VITAMINS', 'ANTI-AGE FOODS'.
He is married with Children .

EBE-TAS PUBLISHERS
ISBN 9780736948
Phn 08023102532